N-Acetylcysteine (NAC)

A Beginner's Quick Start Overview on Its Use Cases, with FAQs

mf

Disclaimer

By reading this disclaimer, you are accepting the terms of the disclaimer in full. If you disagree with this disclaimer, please do not read the guide.

All of the content within this guide is provided for informational and educational purposes only, and should not be accepted as independent medical or other professional advice. The author is not a doctor, physician, nurse, mental health provider, or registered nutritionist/dietician. Therefore, using and reading this guide does not establish any form of a physician-patient relationship.

Always consult with a physician or another qualified health provider with any issues or questions you might have regarding any sort of medical condition. Do not ever disregard any qualified professional medical advice or delay seeking that advice because of anything you have read in this guide. The information in this guide is not intended to be any sort of medical advice and should not be used in lieu of any medical advice by a licensed and qualified medical professional.

Where applicable, persons shown in the cover images are stock photography models and the publisher has obtained the rights to use the images through license agreements with third-party stock image companies.

Table of Contents

Introduction 7

What Is N-Acetylcysteine (NAC)? 9

How Does it Work? 9

Benefits of N-Acetylcysteine (NAC) 10

Different Forms of N-Acetylcysteine (NAC) 14

Current and Past Research on N-Acetylcysteine (NAC) 17

Use Cases of N-Acetylcysteine (NAC) 19

Pros and Cons 26

Advantages of Supplementing N-Acetylcysteine (NAC) 26

Disadvantages of N-Acetylcysteine (NAC) 29

Potential Side Effects 31

Recommended Dosage and Usage 34

Step-by-Step Guide to Get Started With N-Acetylcysteine (NAC) 36

Precautions for N-Acetylcysteine (NAC) 39

Who should not take N-Acetylcysteine (NAC)? 42

Conclusion 46

FAQs 49

References and Helpful Links 51

Introduction

Are you tired of feeling sluggish and fatigued? Do you often find yourself falling prey to frequent illnesses? N-Acetylcysteine may be the answer you've been searching for. Read on to discover how this remarkable antioxidant can revolutionize your health and well-being.

Did you know that N-Acetylcysteine has been extensively studied for its potent antioxidant properties? Not only does it neutralize harmful free radicals, but it also plays a crucial role in replenishing cellular glutathione levels – the body's master antioxidant. But that's not all; NAC's benefits extend beyond its antioxidant capabilities. From promoting respiratory health to supporting mental clarity, there's a wealth of research backing up its incredible potential.

Imagine having a robust immune system that effortlessly fends off infections. Envision enhanced detoxification and liver support to keep your body functioning optimally. Picture experiencing improved cognitive function, leading to sharper focus and better memory. These are just a few of the benefits that N-Acetylcysteine can offer. By incorporating this powerful antioxidant into your daily regimen, you can take control of your health and experience a renewed sense of vitality.

In this guide, we will talk about the following:

- What is N-Acetylcysteine (NAC)?
- How Does It Work?
- Health Benefits, Different Types, and Forms of N-Acetylcysteine (NAC)
- Use Cases
- Pros and Cons
- Potential Side Effects
- Recommended Dosage and Usage
- Step Guide to Get Started with NAC and Precautions for NAC
- Who Should Not Take N-Acetylcysteine (NAC)

Ready to embark on a journey towards better health and well-being? Stay tuned as we delve deeper into the world of N-Acetylcysteine. In the upcoming sections, we will explore its origins, the science behind its effectiveness, and its diverse applications in various health conditions. Get ready to unlock the full potential of this remarkable antioxidant and discover how it can revolutionize your life.

What Is N-Acetylcysteine (NAC)?

N-Acetylcysteine, also known as NAC for short, is an amino acid that has been chemically altered. It is an extremely powerful antioxidant that can eliminate dangerous free radicals and replace glutathione levels in the body, which is the primary antioxidant in the body. NAC has been recognized for a long time for its powerful therapeutic powers, and research suggests that it may have a wide range of potentially beneficial effects on a variety of health disorders.

NAC was initially developed and granted approval for use in medicine in the late 1960s, which is when its usage in medicine began. NAC has been the subject of increased research over the years, which has led to the discovery of its various therapeutic applications as well as knowledge of its methods of action.

How Does it Work?

The efficiency of NAC can be ascribed to the compound's capacity to protect cells from oxidative damage caused by free radicals. NAC can perform its function as an antioxidant by combining with and nullifying reactive oxygen species (ROS), which are toxic chemicals that are capable of causing damage to cells, tissues, and DNA.

In addition to this, glutathione, a powerful antioxidant that is created naturally in the body, is restored to depleted cellular levels when NAC is taken. As a result of age-related reductions in glutathione levels, which are responsible for shielding cells from the oxidative and free radical damage that might occur, taking a NAC supplement becomes increasingly vital.

NAC is effective because it modulates some different metabolic pathways in the body. It has been demonstrated that it interacts with receptors involved in inflammatory processes, cell signaling processes, and neurotransmission, all of which play a role in one's general health and sense of well-being.

Benefits of N-Acetylcysteine (NAC)

NAC has been extensively studied for its therapeutic capabilities, with research suggesting it may have a wide range of potential benefits in various health conditions. Below are just some of the many benefits that NAC can offer:

Replenishing antioxidants

N-Acetylcysteine (NAC) is a potent antioxidant that restores glutathione levels in the body. Glutathione, an essential molecule, protects cells from oxidative stress. NAC strengthens the body's natural antioxidant defenses, reducing damage caused by free radicals to cells and tissues.

This antioxidant promotes lung function, supports the immune system, and aids liver detoxification. It benefits those facing oxidative stress, like individuals exposed to pollutants or chronic infections, by deactivating harmful compounds. Taking NAC supplements daily promotes optimal cellular health and counteracts the negative effects of oxidative stress.

Brain nourishment

N-Acetylcysteine (NAC) has positive effects on brain health. It enhances cognitive function, and memory, and stimulates nerve cell growth. NAC also reduces brain inflammation, protecting against oxidative stress caused by free radicals. Unlock its potential by including NAC in your daily routine for enhanced cognitive performance, sharper concentration, improved memory, and increased vitality.

Respiratory conditions

N-Acetylcysteine (NAC) has long been used to treat respiratory disorders like bronchitis and asthma. It reduces lung inflammation, easing symptoms such as wheezing, coughing, and breathlessness. NAC also thins mucus, aiding its removal from the body.

Moreover, NAC lowers oxidative stress in the lungs, shielding them from further damage. It is a beneficial dietary supplement for individuals with persistent respiratory disorders like cystic fibrosis or COPD, as well as those frequently exposed to environmental toxins.

Immune function

N-Acetylcysteine (NAC) has various positive effects on the immune system, including increased infection and boosted immunity. It promotes the production of white blood cells, the body's natural defense against bacteria and viruses, thus explaining its effectiveness.

Moreover, NAC may help reduce inflammation, further strengthening the immune system and defending against infection. Taking a consistent NAC supplement can enhance the body's natural defenses and overall immune performance, making it a valuable dietary supplement for maintaining health and preventing illness.

Balancing hormones

N-Acetylcysteine (NAC) can positively impact hormonal balance by influencing estrogen and androgen behavior. These hormones regulate processes like growth, development, and reproduction. NAC also boosts melatonin production, regulates sleep patterns, and reduces cortisol levels, which respond to stress.

Regular NAC supplementation can help maintain hormonal balance, alleviating symptoms like exhaustion, irritability, and weight gain. It's an effective supplement for achieving optimal health and well-being.

Insulin sensitivity

N-Acetylcysteine (NAC) has been studied for its potential benefits in managing diabetes. It can help lower insulin resistance, a condition where the body doesn't properly utilize insulin to convert glucose into energy.

This can lead to type 2 diabetes. NAC stimulates enzymes and proteins involved in glucose metabolism, reducing blood glucose levels. It also reduces inflammation, associated with metabolic illnesses like diabetes and obesity. NAC is a beneficial supplement for improving insulin sensitivity and regulating blood sugar levels.

In general, taking NAC supplements regularly can help protect cells from damage caused by oxidative stress and lower the risk of developing chronic diseases such as cancer and heart disease. Because of this, it is an effective dietary supplement for people who are interested in improving their general health and well-being.

Different Forms of
N-Acetylcysteine (NAC)

There are different forms of N-Acetylcysteine (NAC) available on the market. Some common forms include:

Oral capsules

Supplementation with N-Acetylcysteine (NAC) is most commonly taken in the form of capsules for oral consumption. They are convenient to take because they are available in tablet or capsule form, which makes it easier for the digestive system to absorb them. The use of NAC capsules has the benefit of delivering a uniform dose, which makes it much simpler to keep track of how much NAC is being used.

In addition, the efficacy and safety of ingesting NAC capsules orally are well-established in scientific research as well as in actual usage in the real world. Individuals who are looking for the therapeutic benefits of NAC typically choose to supplement their diet with NAC capsules because of all of these advantages. It is no wonder that NAC capsules continue to be the favored choice.

Effervescent tablets

Consumers who have trouble swallowing capsules or who choose a more convenient consumption technique have shown a significant increase in interest in effervescent NAC tablet options. These tablets, when mixed with water, provide a carbonated beverage that is not only simple to consume but also quite delightful.

The robust antioxidant qualities of NAC supplements, as well as their capacity to improve respiratory health, have made them quite popular. Effervescent NAC tablets provide a novel method to supplement one's diet with this vital ingredient and are designed to be simple to adapt into one's daily routine to offer continuous support for one's health.

Powder

The powdered version of N-acetylcysteine, also known as NAC, is a handy supplement that may be easily combined with liquids such as water or other beverages. Powdered NAC, in contrast to other types of supplements such as capsules or tablets, can have its dosage readily adjusted to meet the requirements of a particular individual. In addition, some people find that taking alternative forms of NAC, such as capsules or liquid, results in the supplement having a disagreeable flavor. Mixing NAC powder with a beverage can help cover this taste.

The powdered form of NAC has the potential to be less stable than other forms of the supplement. Because of this, it must be kept in a dark, cold, and dry location away from sources of light and heat to preserve its effectiveness. In general, powdered NAC is a form of supplement that is convenient and adaptable, making it an ideal choice for individuals who favor a liquid consistency or who need to change their dosage.

Intravenous (IV) solution

N-Acetylcysteine (NAC), when given intravenously, can be utilized for the treatment of particular illnesses as well as urgent medical situations. Because the body can absorb this type of NAC more quickly, it is possible to experience speedier alleviation and treatment. Patients in hospitals and other medical facilities frequently get intravenous NAC for the treatment of a variety of illnesses, including liver failure, acetaminophen overdose, respiratory distress, and others.

In addition to this, it is frequently utilized in emergency rooms to expeditiously treat individuals who are suffering from acute liver failure. Due to the possibility of it causing unwanted effects, it must be provided with extreme caution and under the watchful eye of a physician even if it is an effective therapeutic option. The administration of NAC via the intravenous route is an essential component of the provision of this beneficial medication to patients who are in need.

It is essential to take the product by the recommendations for the appropriate dosage that is printed on the product packaging or as directed by a healthcare practitioner.

Current and Past Research on N-Acetylcysteine (NAC)

N-Acetylcysteine (NAC) is one of the most widely studied supplements due to its potential for treating various illnesses and medical conditions. Recent research has been looking into the therapeutic uses of this supplement, such as its potential use in the treatment of respiratory infections, mental health conditions, addiction, cancer, and more. In addition to this, research is also being conducted to explore the potential of NAC as a protective agent against oxidative stress, which is believed to contribute to the development of chronic diseases.

In terms of mental health and addiction, recent research has suggested that supplementing with NAC may help reduce symptoms associated with anxiety, depression, obsessive-compulsive disorder (OCD), post-traumatic stress disorder (PTSD), and addiction. Research has also suggested that NAC may be beneficial in the treatment of other illnesses such as chronic fatigue syndrome, autism spectrum disorders, and Alzheimer's disease.

In terms of cancer, research is still ongoing to explore if supplementing with NAC could help reduce the risk of developing certain forms of this illness. Thus far, research has suggested that supplementing with NAC may help reduce the risk of certain types of cancer such as lung and prostate.

Emerging evidence suggests that supplementing with NAC may offer significant benefits to individuals with respiratory conditions like asthma and cystic fibrosis. Research indicates that NAC has the potential to effectively treat these conditions by alleviating symptoms and promoting better respiratory health.

N-Acetylcysteine (NAC) is a supplement that has been extensively studied in terms of its various therapeutic benefits. With the growing body of evidence supporting its use, more individuals are beginning to explore the potential of using this supplement for various purposes such as improving mental health, fighting addiction, and reducing the risk of cancer.

It is important to remember that while NAC has been proven to be effective in some areas, more research is still needed to fully understand all of its potential uses and benefits. As always, individuals should consult with their healthcare provider before taking any supplement or making any changes to their diet or lifestyle.

Use Cases of N-Acetylcysteine (NAC)

N-Acetylcysteine (NAC) has a wide range of potential uses, from improving respiratory health to aiding in diabetes management. It is most commonly used to alleviate symptoms related to oxidative stress and certain chronic conditions. Below are some common use cases for NAC supplementation:

Treatment for Acetaminophen Overdose

N-acetylcysteine, often known as NAC, is a medication that is widely acknowledged as being beneficial in the event that someone has overdosed on acetaminophen, also known as Tylenol. NAC serves as an antidote by restoring levels of glutathione, a powerful antioxidant that is lost when an individual consumes an excessive amount of the drug. Glutathione is an essential component in the body's defense against the harmful metabolites that are generated when there is an abundance of acetaminophen.

NAC helps prevent liver damage, which can be a significant result of taking an excessive amount of acetaminophen. It does this by restoring glutathione levels in the body. The usefulness of NAC has been demonstrated in clinical tests, and it can be given either orally or intravenously. Medical recommendations have endorsed the use of this supplement. In circumstances when an overdose of acetaminophen may have occurred, it is critical to seek medical assistance as soon as possible.

Respiratory Conditions

N-acetylcysteine has shown promise as a potential treatment for a variety of respiratory disorders. It has been demonstrated to be effective in easing mucus congestion, enhancing lung function, and reducing the severity of symptoms. Because of the mucolytic qualities of NAC, mucus can be broken down and thinned, making it simpler to remove mucus from the airways.

Patients suffering from illnesses such as chronic obstructive pulmonary disease (also known as COPD), asthma, and cystic fibrosis may gain some benefit from this. In addition, the antioxidant capabilities of NAC may assist in lowering inflammation in the airways and providing protection against the damaging effects of oxidative stress. NAC has potential as a supplemental treatment for respiratory diseases, while additional research is required to completely appreciate its effectiveness.

Antioxidant Support

N-acetylcysteine (NAC) serves as a vital component in the production of glutathione, a powerful antioxidant found naturally in the body. Glutathione plays a crucial role in protecting cells from oxidative stress caused by free radicals, which can damage DNA, proteins, and lipids. By enhancing glutathione levels, NAC reinforces the body's defense mechanisms against oxidative stress and helps maintain cellular health. This antioxidant support provided by NAC has been linked to various health benefits.

Mental Health Support

N-acetylcysteine has been found to have the potential as a therapeutic adjunct for a variety of mental health disorders. According to research, NAC may be beneficial for patients suffering from depression, bipolar illness, and addiction. It is possible that the therapeutic effects of NAC are due, in part, to its capacity to modulate neurotransmitters like glutamate and regulate oxidative stress.

NAC may be able to help reduce inflammation in the brain and support optimum neuronal function by working to lessen the effects of oxidative stress and bolster the antioxidant capabilities of the body. Even though additional research is required to fully understand its mechanisms and effectiveness, NAC is a viable option for mental health support and may complement other treatment approaches. This is despite the fact that more research is required.

Hormonal Balance

N-acetylcysteine (NAC) has shown promising effects in promoting hormonal balance, especially in conditions like polycystic ovary syndrome (PCOS). PCOS is characterized by hormonal imbalances, insulin resistance, and fertility issues. NAC's ability to enhance glutathione levels, reduce oxidative stress, and improve insulin sensitivity makes it beneficial in managing PCOS.

By reducing insulin resistance, NAC can help regulate hormone levels, restore menstrual regularity, and improve ovulation. Additionally, NAC's antioxidant properties may reduce inflammation and oxidative stress associated with PCOS. While further research is needed, NAC holds potential as a natural intervention for restoring hormonal balance and improving fertility outcomes in individuals with PCOS.

Cancer Prevention

N-acetylcysteine is recognized for the antioxidant characteristics that it possesses, and there is a possibility that it could have a role in the prevention of cancer. Damage to cells and even a possible contribution to the development of cancer can be caused by free radicals. NAC helps protect cells from oxidative stress and DNA damage by removing potentially dangerous free radicals from the cell's environment.

In addition, NAC helps to maintain cellular integrity and overall health by stimulating the production of glutathione, a potent antioxidant that plays a role in the elimination of toxins and the preservation of cellular structure. NAC's capacity to battle oxidative stress implies that it may have the potential as a beneficial adjunct in reducing the risk of cancer formation. However, additional research is required to establish a conclusive link between NAC and the prevention of cancer.

Protection against Hepato- and Nephrotoxicity

N-acetylcysteine has demonstrated that it has the potential to protect the liver and kidneys against the toxicity that is caused by other chemicals. This is accomplished by restoring depleted levels of glutathione, which is an essential antioxidant that plays a role in the detoxification process. Because of its capacity to stimulate glutathione production, NAC contributes to the process of removing and neutralizing toxins that are harmful to these organs.

NAC works as a shield, minimizing the harmful effects of toxic compounds such as some drugs, toxins, and environmental contaminants. It does this by bolstering the body's natural defenses and defense mechanisms against attack. Because of this protective role, NAC is a useful ally in the process of maintaining the health and function of the liver and kidneys, which are key organs that are essential for maintaining general health.

Neurodegenerative Conditions

The treatment of neurodegenerative disorders including Alzheimer's disease and Parkinson's disease may benefit from the administration of N-acetylcysteine, also known as NAC. According to the findings of several studies, NAC may be able to provide numerous benefits in these cases. It has shown some promise in preventing damage to neurons, lowering inflammation in the brain, and improving antioxidant defenses.

It is possible that NAC can help slow down the evolution of neurodegenerative disorders including Parkinson's disease and Alzheimer's disease by altering the action of neurotransmitters and lowering oxidative stress. NAC is a possible path for supporting persons who are living with neurodegenerative conditions such as Alzheimer's disease, Parkinson's disease, and other neurodegenerative conditions; however, additional research is required to fully understand its mechanisms and usefulness.

N-Acetylcysteine (NAC) is a supplement with numerous potential applications in health and wellness. It has been linked to providing support for various respiratory conditions, mental health issues, hormonal imbalances, cancer prevention, and neurodegenerative diseases. Its ability to modulate neurotransmitter activity, reduce inflammation, and protect cells from oxidation offers immense potential in supporting optimal health and well-being. NAC can be a valuable tool for those seeking natural interventions to enhance their overall health.

However, it is important to consult with a healthcare professional before using this supplement as its effects may vary from person to person. With proper guidance, NAC can be an effective complement to existing treatment plans and help restore balance and vitality.

Pros and Cons

Like any supplement, NAC comes with its own set of pros and cons. In this section, we will explore the advantages and disadvantages of supplementing N-Acetylcysteine (NAC), shedding light on the potential benefits it offers as well as the considerations one should keep in mind before incorporating it into their routine.

Advantages of Supplementing N-Acetylcysteine (NAC)

Supplementing with N-Acetylcysteine (NAC) has many potential benefits. Here are some of the main advantages associated with its use:

Non-Invasive

One of the significant advantages of N-Acetylcysteine (NAC) is its non-invasive nature, which makes it a safe and well-tolerated supplement for most individuals, regardless of age or health condition. Unlike certain medications, NAC is known for its minimal risk of serious side effects and does not necessitate special monitoring or extensive medical supervision.

This outstanding safety profile makes NAC an attractive choice for those seeking a natural, gentle, and reliable means to support and enhance their body's overall function and well-being.

Affordability

N-Acetylcysteine (NAC) supplements are considered to be one of the most affordable solutions available in the supplement market, making it a financially prudent choice for persons who are interested in improving their general health.

This is especially true when compared to other supplements that are typically used for purposes that are analogous to those of this one. Because of the low price at which it may be purchased, NAC continues to be a well-liked choice among individuals who are interested in preserving their health without breaking the budget.

Versatility

N-Acetylcysteine (NAC) is a highly versatile supplement that has shown promising potential in addressing a wide range of health issues. Extensive research has been conducted on its efficacy, and it has demonstrated positive effects in various conditions, including addiction recovery, stroke prevention, and even mental health support. With such a diverse spectrum of potential benefits, NAC emerges as an appealing choice for individuals seeking a comprehensive and multi-purpose supplement to enhance their overall well-being.

Well-Tolerated

N-Acetylcysteine (NAC) has the benefit of being well-tolerated by the vast majority of people and causing just a small amount of adverse effects when taken in acceptable amounts. This is because it can readily convert into glutathione, which is a potent antioxidant found within the body. NAC is less likely to produce allergic reactions than other synthetic substances because it is derived from an amino acid that occurs naturally in the body. Because of this, it is a safe choice for people who are allergic to or sensitive to the ingredients in other supplements.

Individuals who are interested in improving their health may find that using NAC (N-Acetyl Cysteine) dietary supplements offers several benefits that make this choice a tempting one. However, before beginning a new supplement routine, it is essential to discuss the supplement with a qualified medical practitioner to confirm that the supplement is appropriate for the individual's specific requirements and existing health concerns. A holistic strategy for health and wellness may benefit from the addition of NAC supplementation if this is done correctly.

Disadvantages of N-Acetylcysteine (NAC)

Although there are many advantages associated with supplementing N-Acetylcysteine (NAC), there are also some potential drawbacks to consider. These include;

Not suitable for everyone

Because it has the potential to interact with some other medical problems and medications, N-Acetylcysteine, or NAC, is not appropriate for everyone to take. NAC should be used with caution or only under the supervision of a healthcare expert by individuals who suffer from asthma, blood disorders, liver illness, or renal disease.

In addition, there is a possibility that NAC will interact negatively with blood-thinning medications, nitroglycerin, and chemotherapy treatments. Before taking NAC as a supplement, it is imperative to consult a physician to ensure that you won't have any negative side effects.

Lack of regulation

Because there are no regulations in place, it can be difficult to make sure that N-acetylcysteine (NAC) supplements have the right amount of the active component and that it is present in a consistent manner throughout the product. Ineffective manufacturing techniques may also produce contamination, which may cause undesirable side effects or render treatment ineffective.

Before making a purchase, customers looking to buy NAC supplements have to exercise extreme caution and thoroughly investigate the reputation of the producer. In general, the absence of regulations for dietary supplements such as NAC underscores the significance of monitoring and education for consumers.

Limited scientific evidence

N-Acetylcysteine (NAC) does have some drawbacks, one of which is that although being researched for a variety of potentially beneficial effects on health, not all claims are supported by solid scientific data. Because of the lack of proof, there are questions about whether or not NAC is effective and safe for treating certain illnesses. Therefore, before employing NAC as a medication, it is vital to conduct additional research into each prospective health benefit to validate both its efficacy and safety.

To ensure that the medicine is used safely, it is necessary to take into account not only the appropriate dosage and time but also any possible interactions with other medications. Those who are thinking about taking NAC as a treatment need to give careful attention to the fact that there is insufficient scientific data to support the claims that NAC has beneficial effects on one's health.

N-Acetylcysteine (NAC) supplements may have certain possible downsides; nevertheless, the benefits of taking these supplements can frequently outweigh these potential issues. Before beginning a new supplement regimen, it is essential to get advice from a qualified medical practitioner to guarantee that the supplement will meet the specific requirements of the individual as well as their current state of health. A holistic strategy for health and wellbeing can benefit from the addition of NAC supplementation, provided that its use is supervised by a trained professional.

Potential Side Effects

In general, N-Acetylcysteine (NAC) is well-tolerated and has minimal side effects. Some of the most common side effects associated with its use include;

Gastrointestinal upset

When taken in supplement form, N-acetylcysteine (NAC) has the potential to cause gastrointestinal distress, which can manifest itself in the form of abdominal pain, nausea, vomiting, or diarrhea in some people. It is recommended that patients begin treatment with lower doses, and then gradually increase the amount of medication they take based on how well it is tolerated.

Taking such precautions may assist to reduce the likelihood of experiencing unpleasant effects and ensure that NAC supplementation is done in a manner that is both safe and effective. However, it is critical to seek the advice of a qualified medical practitioner without delay if you have any severe symptoms or bad reactions. Doing so will help you avoid any potential injury or consequences.

Headache

N-Acetylcysteine (NAC) is a supplement that has a wide range of applications due to its many curative properties. On the other hand, a lot of people report that it gives them headaches. This happens because NAC alters the amounts of neurotransmitters in the brain, which may produce headaches if they are severe enough. Fortunately, taking NAC with food has been shown to help reduce both the severity and the frequency of headaches of this type.

Despite this, it is essential to keep a close eye on the symptoms and get medical help if the headache gets worse or continues for more than a few days. It is well known that NAC is a supplement that has a lot of untapped potential, but to get the most out of it, you need to be aware of any potential adverse reactions.

Rashes or itching

N-Acetylcysteine (NAC)has some potential adverse effects, the most common of which is itching or rashes on the skin. It is important to treat this side effect carefully because it may be an indication of an allergic reaction, although the likelihood of experiencing it is low.

It is recommended that a person stop using NAC and seek medical treatment if they get rashes or itching on their skin as a side effect of using the supplement. It is also essential to keep in mind that the severity of an allergic reaction to NAC can vary greatly from one individual to the next, with some people exhibiting only minor symptoms while others exhibit severe reactions. Because of this, it is extremely important to keep an eye out for any peculiar symptoms and get medical help if it is required.

Although N-Acetylcysteine (NAC) is generally well tolerated, certain people can experience adverse effects from its use. It is essential to keep a close eye out for any possible adverse effects and to stop using the product if those effects become apparent. Before beginning any new supplement routine, it is strongly suggested that you discuss your plans with a qualified medical practitioner.

Recommended Dosage and Usage

It is necessary to consult with a knowledgeable medical professional regarding the amount of N-acetylcysteine (NAC) that has to be consumed as well as the manner in which it ought to be utilized. However, particular dose information should be discussed with a medical practitioner, and the suggested daily amount might range anywhere from 600 to 1,200 mg. According to the findings of one research trial, this particular dose range may be useful in treating the condition at hand. In addition, the recommended daily dosage ranges from 600 mg up to 1,200 milligrams for the use of this substance.

However, because the FDA does not regulate NAC supplements, it is crucial to select a brand that has a solid reputation and adheres to the dosage requirements that come with the product. This is especially important because the FDA does not monitor NAC supplements. NAC is generally well tolerated when administered in quantities of 1,200 mg twice daily or lower.

However, at these dosages, unusual adverse effects could potentially manifest themselves. It is essential to take this into consideration. When taking any dietary supplement, it is necessary to take into consideration one's specific health concerns and seek the opinion of a knowledgeable medical practitioner regarding one's ideal dosage. This is the case regardless of whatever supplement one chooses to take.

Step-by-Step Guide to Get Started With N-Acetylcysteine (NAC)

Supplementing with N-Acetylcysteine (NAC) can be beneficial for many health conditions, but it is important to consult with a healthcare provider before starting any supplement regimen. Here are the steps you should take to get started with N-Acetylcysteine (NAC):

Step 1: Consult with a healthcare professional

It is essential to confer with a trained medical expert before beginning the use of any new supplement regimen, including N-Acetylcysteine (NAC), because of the risks associated with doing so. When you do this, you increase the likelihood that your specific health requirements will be taken into account, and you also increase the likelihood that any potential drug interactions you may be experiencing will be thoroughly examined.

In addition, a healthcare professional can provide customized dosage recommendations that are matched to your particular circumstances, maximizing the efficiency and safety of your journey with dietary supplements. Keep in mind that consulting with knowledgeable professionals is an essential step toward arriving at well-informed decisions regarding your health and well-being.

Step 2: Choose a reputable product

When looking for an N-acetylcysteine (NAC) supplement, it is essential to find a brand that has a solid reputation and in which you can have complete confidence. Look for items that not only conform to tight production requirements but also undergo rigorous third-party testing to ensure their quality and purity.

Checking for certifications such as Good Manufacturing Practices (GMP), which assure that the supplement is manufactured in a facility that complies with stringent quality control methods, is one approach to make sure this is the case. Another option to make sure this is the case is to ask the manufacturer about it. You may have the peace of mind that the NAC supplement you purchase is of the best quality and will provide you with the benefits you desire if you give these criteria priority and make them your top priorities.

Step 3: Follow recommended dosage instructions

After speaking with a qualified medical practitioner and acquiring a trustworthy N-Acetylcysteine (NAC) supplement, it is essential to adhere to the dosage instructions that are provided by the manufacturer. The recommended dosage ranges from 600 to 1,200 milligrams per day, but this can change according to the specific requirements of the individual as well as their current state of health. It is essential to make sure that you take the dietary supplement at the frequency recommended by your doctor, whether that be once or twice a day.

Including it in your daily routine consistently is essential if you want to get the full benefits of doing so. You may guarantee that you are receiving the appropriate quantity of NAC to support your health and well-being by adhering to the suggested dose guidelines and following them to the letter. Keep in mind that you should always seek the specialized guidance of a healthcare professional to receive recommendations that are tailored to your unique requirements.

By adhering to these guidelines, you will be able to begin using N-Acetylcysteine (NAC) supplements in a risk-free manner and take advantage of the supplement's many potential health benefits. In addition to this, it is essential to keep a close eye on any symptoms that may develop and to stop using the product if necessary.

Precautions for N-Acetylcysteine (NAC)

Monitor side effects

It is necessary to keep a close eye out for any potential adverse reactions when taking N-Acetylcysteine (NAC) supplements. Even though NAC is usually considered to be safe, some people may develop gastrointestinal distress after taking it. This may include nausea, vomiting, or diarrhea. In addition, there is a possibility that low zinc and copper levels could result from using NAC for an extended period.

Before beginning to take NAC as a supplement, it is critical to discuss the matter with a qualified medical professional. This will help ensure that you do not have any negative side effects. In addition, it is extremely important to adhere to the dosage that is prescribed, as taking excessive amounts of NAC may harm the liver or make asthma symptoms worse. Last but not least, if you experience any unanticipated symptoms or allergic reactions while using NAC, such as respiratory distress or a rash on your skin, you should immediately stop using it and seek medical treatment.

Check for drug interactions

When an individual takes N-Acetylcysteine (NAC) as a dietary supplement, there is always the possibility that it will interact negatively with one or more of the medications that they are already taking. Before beginning treatment with NAC, it is critical to discuss the medication with a qualified medical professional to eliminate the risk of any potentially adverse interactions. When used at the same time as NAC, certain drugs, such as nitroglycerin, could have their effectiveness diminished.

In addition, the use of NAC in conjunction with some drugs, such as carbamazepine or nitroprusside, has the potential to bring the patient's blood pressure down. Before beginning any supplement regimen that includes NAC, it is essential to be aware of any potential interactions and to discuss them with a healthcare provider.

Pregnancy and breastfeeding

When contemplating whether or not to take a supplement containing N-acetylcysteine (NAC), pregnant women and mothers who are breastfeeding are urged to exercise extreme caution. Although NAC is thought to be safe for the vast majority of people, it is extremely important to seek the advice of a qualified medical practitioner before using it while pregnant or nursing a child.

The reason for this is that the safety profile of NAC during these phases has not been fully explored, and the potential effects that it could have on the developing fetus or newborns are yet unknown. Therefore, it is best to err on the side of caution and refrain from using NAC unless under the close supervision of a qualified medical professional.

Do not exceed recommended dosage

It is essential to follow the suggested dosage instructions for N-Acetylcysteine (NAC) if you want to avoid any potential health risks and get the most out of the NAC's possible positive effects on your health. It is extremely important to only take the dose that has been recommended by the doctor because exceeding the prescribed amount can result in unpleasant side effects. By adhering to these rules, you will be able to comfortably use NAC in your daily supplement regimen and maybe take advantage of its multiple beneficial effects on your health.

N-Acetylcysteine (NAC), when ingested by the instructions of a trained professional, has the potential to be an advantageous component of a holistic approach to health and wellness. Before beginning to take this supplement, it is essential to take into account the warnings and possible drug interactions that have been presented previously. Before beginning any new routine, you must speak with a healthcare professional regarding any dietary supplements.

Who should not take N-Acetylcysteine (NAC)?

Certain individuals should not take N-Acetylcysteine (NAC) due to potential risks and contraindications. Here are some considerations for who should not take N-Acetylcysteine:

Nitroglycerin use

People who are already treating themselves medically with nitroglycerin, whether in the form of tablets, patches, or lotions, should steer clear of using N-Acetylcysteine, which is more commonly referred to as NAC. This combination has the potential to bring about a significant reduction in blood pressure, which in turn has the potential to bring about headaches and other potential health hazards. Because of this, considerable caution needs to be given when administering these two medications at the same time, and individuals should always consult their healthcare expert prior to making use of NAC.

Nitroglycerin is commonly used to treat persistent chest discomfort, despite the fact that NAC has been discovered to provide a variety of health benefits, including enhancing antioxidant levels, improving liver function, and reducing inflammation. Nitroglycerin is employed in a variety of settings. It is crucial to make an educated decision before taking both of these medications at the same time. This should be done after carefully assessing the potential benefits of doing so as well as the potential risks of doing so.

Children

N-acetylcysteine is never to be given to a child unless it is being closely monitored by a trained medical practitioner. This is a strict rule. This is due to the fact that children may have different dose requirements than adults, and the study regarding the efficacy and safety of NAC in children has not been conducted to a sufficient level. In addition to this, it is possible that the dosage requirements for adults and children will be very different from one another. Additionally, children may be more susceptible to the adverse effects of the medicine, such as allergic reactions.

It is absolutely necessary to have a conversation about the therapy with a trained medical professional before administering NAC to youngsters. The medical practitioner will be able to determine whether the potential benefits of the medication outweigh the hazards that are connected with using it. It is of the utmost importance to follow the instructions given by the physician regarding the dosage as well as the length of time that the medication should be administered.

Hypersensitivity reactions

It is essential to point out that people who have ever had any kind of hypersensitive reaction to N-Acetylcysteine (NAC) in the past should not drink it. This recommendation applies to both current and former users. NAC is a powerful antioxidant that is frequently recommended for a wide range of medical issues. On the other hand, the medicine may produce an instant and severe response in a person who has a history of having allergic responses to it.

Reactions caused by hypersensitivity can range from being quite harmless to being potentially fatal. Because of this, it is extremely important to steer clear of NAC if a person has ever experienced an unpleasant reaction in the past to avoid any potential injury. Before beginning treatment with this drug, it is strongly recommended that you discuss your condition with a medical expert. Doing so will help you avoid any unintended effects.

Before beginning the use of any new dietary supplement or drug, including N-Acetylcysteine, it is of the greatest significance to check with a certified healthcare expert, such as a doctor or pharmacist. This is especially important if you are pregnant or nursing.

This preventative measure is essential to ensuring that the supplement or drug is not only risk-free but also appropriate for your current state of health. This involves taking into account the possibility of adverse interactions with any medications you are already taking, as well as any allergies or other health conditions that you may have. You will be able to make educated decisions regarding your healthcare if you seek the help of professionals. These decisions will allow you to maximize the potential advantages while reducing any potential hazards.

Conclusion

You've reached the end of your N-Acetylcysteine (NAC) Guide, and what a journey it has been! Congratulations on expanding your knowledge about this incredible compound. As you wrap up this guide, let's recap some key insights and leave you feeling inspired to incorporate NAC into your life.

We've covered a lot of ground in this tutorial when it comes to the outstanding advantages that N-acetylcysteine possesses. NAC is a useful and efficient supplement for a variety of reasons, including the high antioxidant qualities it possesses and its capacity to improve respiratory health. NAC helps protect our cells from the damaging effects of oxidative stress by increasing the amount of glutathione in our bodies. This has a positive impact on our overall health.

NAC, however, does not stop there. research reveals that it can treat symptoms of disorders such as depression, anxiety, and obsessive-compulsive disorder. It has shown promise in promoting mental health, and this research implies that it has the potential to do so. Because of its ability to modify neurotransmitter levels as well as reduce inflammation, it is an extremely useful tool for the maintenance of a healthy brain.

N-Acetylcysteine has been shown to have remarkable promise in the treatment of substance dependence, in addition to the positive effects it has on mental health. NAC helps reduce cravings and minimize withdrawal symptoms by restoring glutathione levels and boosting detoxification. These effects are achieved through the promotion of detoxification. This demonstrates the ground-breaking character of the compound by providing those seeking recovery with fresh opportunities and opening up new avenues of inquiry.

Therefore, how exactly can you incorporate N-acetylcysteine into your everyday routine? To begin, it is recommended that you seek the advice of a qualified medical practitioner to ascertain the correct dosage and make certain that it is suitable for your requirements. NAC can be a helpful ally for you whether you are wanting to improve your physical well-being, support your mental health, or get assistance in recovering from an addiction.

Always keep in mind that reliability is essential. It is essential to include N-acetylcysteine in your routine and to give it enough time to work its wonders before doing so. Maintaining your NAC regimen consistently over time can, even though individual results may vary, result in significant benefits in the long term.

When using any kind of supplement, it is necessary to think about the possible adverse effects and interactions. Be sure to address any preexisting medical conditions as well as any medications that you are currently taking with a qualified medical expert. They will give you advice that is suited to your particular situation, which will ensure that your time spent with NAC is productive and risk-free.

As you come to the end of this guide, allow the information you've received to motivate you to put what you've learned into practice. N-Acetylcysteine holds the key to a world of wellness; all you need to do is embrace its potential. Keep in mind that you hold the power to improve your health and well-being and that taking NAC may prove to be an extremely helpful tool on your road.

Having gained this new knowledge, it is time to put it to use and make the most of the benefits that N-acetylcysteine has to offer. Get the most out of its antioxidant power, take care of your mental health, and make the most of its ability to aid in the recovery from addiction. There is no limit to the possibilities, and the journey to a happier and healthier life can begin at any time.

FAQs

What is N-Acetylcysteine (NAC)?

N-Acetylcysteine (NAC) is a supplement derived from the amino acid L-cysteine. It has various uses and is an FDA-approved drug.

What are the benefits of taking NAC?

NAC has been associated with several potential health benefits, including antioxidant support, respiratory health support, liver detoxification support, and mental health support.

How should NAC be taken?

NAC should be taken either 30 minutes before or two hours after eating to avoid competition with protein for absorption. It is important to follow the recommended dosage instructions provided by the manufacturer or healthcare provider.

Are there any side effects of NAC?

NAC can cause side effects such as dry mouth, nausea, vomiting, diarrhea, and an unpleasant odor. It is important to consult with a healthcare provider if you experience any severe or persistent side effects.

Is NAC safe during pregnancy and breastfeeding?

Limited research is available on the safety of NAC during pregnancy and breastfeeding. It is recommended to consult with a healthcare provider before using NAC if you are pregnant or breastfeeding.

Can NAC interact with medications?

NAC may interact with certain medications, such as nitroglycerin, ACE inhibitors, and nitroprusside. It is important to inform your healthcare provider about all the medications you are taking to avoid potential interactions.

Are there any precautions or contraindications for taking NAC?

Individuals with asthma, bleeding disorders, or those scheduled for elective surgery may need to avoid NAC. It is advisable to discuss the use of NAC with a healthcare provider if you have any pre-existing medical conditions or if you are planning to undergo surgery.

References and Helpful Links

Ld, A. G. M. R. C. (2023, May 15). What are the Health Benefits of NAC (N-Acetyl Cysteine)? Healthline. https://www.healthline.com/nutrition/nac-benefits#:~:text=High%20blood%20sugar%20and%20obesity,improving%20insulin%20resistance%20(%2023%20).

Sadowska, A., Verbraecken, J., Darquennes, K., & De Backer, W. (2006). Role of N-acetylcysteine in the management of COPD. International Journal of Chronic Obstructive Pulmonary Disease, 1(4), 425–434. https://doi.org/10.2147/copd.2006.1.4.425

Tenório, M. C. D. S., Graciliano, N. G., Moura, F. A., De Oliveira, A. C. M., & Goulart, M. O. F. (2021). N-Acetylcysteine (NAC): Impacts on human health. Antioxidants, 10(6), 967. https://doi.org/10.3390/antiox10060967

Ooi, S. L., Green, R., & Pak, S. C. (2018). N-Acetylcysteine for the Treatment of Psychiatric Disorders: A review of Current evidence. BioMed Research International, 2018, 1–8. https://doi.org/10.1155/2018/2469486

Modglin, L. (2023, March 3). What is NAC (N-Acetyl cysteine) supplement? Forbes Health. https://www.forbes.com/health/body/what-is-nac/

Acetylcysteine (Oral route) precautions - Mayo Clinic. (n.d.).
https://www.mayoclinic.org/drugs-supplements/acetylcysteine-oral-route/
precautions/drg-20311314?p=1#:~:text=Tell%20your%20doctor%20righ
t%20away,or%20unusual%20tiredness%20or%20weakness.

Millea, P. J. (2009, August 1). N-Acetylcysteine: multiple clinical
applications. AAFP.
https://www.aafp.org/pubs/afp/issues/2009/0801/p265.html#:~:text=26-,
Adverse%20Reactions%20and%20Drug%20Interactions,%2C%20epigas
tric%20pain%2C%20and%20constipation.

www.ingramcontent.com/pod-product-compliance
Ingram Content Group UK Ltd.
Pitfield, Milton Keynes, MK11 3LW, UK
UKHW020822011025
8163UKWH00043B/880